The Doctor Said What?

One Man's Victory Over Ulcerative Colitis

Don Makowski

DISCLAIMER

This book details the author's personal experiences with and opinions about Ulcerative Colitis. The author is not a healthcare provider.

The author and publisher are providing this book and its contents on an "as is" basis and make no representations or warranties of any kind with respect to this book or its contents. The author and publisher disclaim all such representations and warranties, including for example warranties of merchantability and healthcare for a particular purpose. In addition, the author and publisher do not represent or warrant that the information accessible via this book is accurate, complete or current.

The statements made about products and services have not been evaluated by the U.S. Food and Drug Administration. They are not intended to diagnose, treat, cure, or prevent any condition or disease. Please consult with your own physician or healthcare specialist regarding the suggestions and recommendations made in this book.

Except as specifically stated in this book, neither the author or publisher, nor any authors, contributors, or other representatives will be liable for damages arising out of or in connection with the use of this book. This is a comprehensive limitation of liability that applies to all damages of any kind, including (without limitation) compensatory; direct, indirect or consequential damages; loss of data, income or profit; loss of or damage to property and claims of third parties.

You understand that this book is not intended as a substitute for consultation with a licensed healthcare practitioner, such as your physician. Before you begin any healthcare program, or change your lifestyle in any way, you will consult your physician or other licensed healthcare practitioner to ensure that you are in good health and that the examples contained in this book will not harm you.

This book provides content related to topics physical and/or mental health issues. As such, use of this book implies your acceptance of this disclaimer.

Thank you!

More than anyone else I would like to thank my wife Suzi for all that she endured through this trying time, for never giving up and always encouraging me to continue to pursue a cure. I spent a lot of money trying this and that and never once did she have a negative word about it. Thank you Suzi for your love and for your kindness. Thank you for your support and encouragement. Michael Hursts' book 'How I Cured Myself of Ulcerative Colitis' was invaluable in my treatment. Thank you Michael and I hope you continue to have good health. Thank you Mom and Dad. I know you suffered watching me suffer. No one should have to watch their child wither away as I did. Thank you to my friends and family. There are too many of you to mention but I appreciate you and love you all. Thank you for being there for me.

Table of Contents

The doctor said what?

He told me that I had Ulcerative Colitis. There was no cure. I would have it for the rest of my life.

Introduction

Hello, my name is Don Makowski and I have decided to share my story to help others understand Ulcerative Colitis and to help those of you who have bowel problems. I am cured now!!! I cured myself with home fecal transplant therapy. You will find my complete experience in this book. I no longer have any symptoms of U.C. The problem with home fecal transplantation is that you have to be very desperate before you can go through with it. I urge you to take care of this before the inflammation gets that bad. You can avoid so much pain and suffering. I offer my story with this in mind.

My experience with the medical community has left some serious scars. I do not carry medical insurance now because I see the system as corrupt. When you have insurance they see you as a dollar sign. There is this idea among doctors that we are defective human beings and that our immune systems are the problem. This is a lie! Our immune systems protect and warn us of problems. If we suppress this system we are inviting trouble.

Ulcerative Colitis exists in my family. Why? It's related to the gut bacteria that we all share and also to our environment and lifestyle. I lost an Aunt to this condition, I have an Uncle, Cousin and Nephew who have had colostomies. I have a younger brother who is on Imuran. This is definitely in the family but that doesn't mean we have defective genes. Fecal transplant therapy has been known about since the fourth century in China! Why has it been lost? Most holistic medicine has been lost since the formation of the AMA in 1847. That's another story and a sad one that I urge you to look into.

A for-profit medical system cannot be trusted. There is no profit in curing sickness; there is no profit in death. There is only profit in keeping people sick. It's shameful but true. I wish you the best of health and hope you can benefit from my story. I also hope that someday the system will change. The internet is a powerful and valuable tool in making this change. Don't just accept what the doctors tell you! Investigate it for yourself. I know it's difficult but I can tell you that I am so very, very happy to have my colon intact. That is a direct result of not giving up and not accepting!

The Dog Gets Sick

My health before U.C. had always been good and I considered myself healthy and strong. My wife called me the dog because I could eat anything. I stayed fit and trim, was active, exercised, played musical instruments, sang, and wrote music. I was happily married and had children and grandchildren. Life was good. I was employed as an injection mold designer and made a decent living.

Tool and Die can be a very demanding profession for the toolmakers, owners, and designers, especially in a small shop environment. I worked at a small tool shop in Erie, PA when I first started to notice a change in my system. This was right after the business had seen much success and had moved to a new facility. I was still healthy and taking daily walks of about a mile long at lunchtime. I noticed that my butt was starting to itch more and more as I walked. It felt wet, like it was leaking, and I usually had to go to the bathroom when I got back. I also noticed that I was going to the bathroom more and that my stools were looser. No big deal. I could live with it. I was a beer drinker too. I didn't drink much liquor, only Coors light. I drank a lot of it on weekends but very little during the week. My wife and I loved to go out drinking and dancing to live rock music every weekend. We had a blast following the local scene!

I was a designer at this shop for six years when the owners saw a downturn in business after 9/11. The pressure started to get to them. I thought that I would always work for them but this was not to be. I was let go one day and was absolutely shocked to find myself unemployed. Luckily there was a tool shop right next door. I had a friend who worked there who told the owners that they would be crazy to not hire me. They did and I even got a raise! This was a stressful time but it was ok. I was still ok.

I had settled into my new position nicely and got along with my new boss, owners, and fellow employees well. The toolmakers there were very helpful and it was a good place to work. After I was there a couple years the owners decided to cut our pay by 10% and to eliminate our overtime. They said they had to do it to remain competitive with the Chinese. That was a huge hit to take and now I was worrying about losing my house. I believe that the stress from this situation was partially responsible for my first flare.

In the fall of 2006 I released my first CD of original music under the name Dee Girard (www.deegirard.com). This was an exciting time for me as I had always wanted to write music. I wrote all the songs, set up a home studio, learned how to use new digital recording equipment, recorded and engineered, played all the instruments and sang, added harmonies and did all the editing on this disc. It was a lot of work and the culmination of a three year project. When my wages were cut I had to sell off all of my musical equipment to pay my mortgage. This was very difficult but I had no other options. We had also planned and paid for a trip to Savannah that summer. About a week before my vacation I started to notice blood in my stools. My first thoughts were that I had cancer now so I might as well just keep it to myself and go and enjoy this one last vacation with my wife before I died. We had a nice time but I was worried and knew I had to face it soon.

After returning from vacation things got steadily worse. I had not told anyone and it was awful keeping this to myself. One Friday afternoon at work I had to go to the bathroom again. I was going 6-10 times per day and I know my fellow employees and boss were wondering what was going on. I sat down and nothing came out but bright red blood. I knew this was not going to resolve itself and it was time to call my family doctor. I made an appointment to see her in a couple weeks. I thought they would want me to go to the ER or want to see me right away but they didn't act like it was a big deal. Really weird! After seeing her and getting the finger probe she told me that there was blood. I knew that already! That's why I was there for the love of god! She set up an appointment for me to see a gastroenterologist and said there was nothing else that could be done at this time. Yup, weird!

I first saw The G.I.'s physician assistant in the late summer of 2007. She asked questions about my bowel habits and about my family history. I told her that I had an aunt that had died of Crohn's disease, an uncle and a cousin who had colostomy bags, a brother, a sister, and a nephew who were diagnosed with UC. I thought that my condition was serious but she said nothing needed to be done yet and that I would need a colonoscopy in about a month. She never asked me about lifestyle and

I never got to see the doctor. I was pretty bad off at that time but had no idea how bad it was going to get. I was having diarrhea 5-6 times a day and losing weight quickly. Finally the day came for me to do the bowel prep. What a horrifying experience that was! After having diarrhea so bad I was now inducing it! I had to stay in the bathroom most of the night and was screaming in agony. I had the colonoscopy and was sent home with no help. I thought that was strange since by looking at me you could tell that I was anemic and looked sick. I called the doctors' office several days later to see what they could do for me but was told that I had to wait for the results of the colonoscopy before they could determine a treatment. The receptionist told me to take some Imodium! The doctor was on vacation! Wow!

I called my G.I. again as they still had not spoken to me about the results of my colonoscopy. He told me that I had Ulcerative Colitis. I would have it for the rest of my life and that I would always be on medication. I couldn't believe it! I felt like my life was over. I asked him if there was anything I could do. Could I change my diet? What about drinking? Should I stop? He was unconcerned about this and just said no, diet had nothing to do with this disease and there was nothing I could do but continue taking Asacol which wasn't making a bit of difference. I cried that day in my bosses' office after that call. I felt absolutely lost. I was a defective human being.

Another week went by and still no help. I made an appointment with a holistic doctor who had treated himself for Crohn's disease. I had one session with this guy, I don't remember his name, but he seemed to know what he was doing. He performed acupuncture on me and sold me some Chinese herbs, vegetable mix and powders all at a cost of nearly $300. I began these as soon as I got home and was now at the point where I could no longer go to work. I took an emergency leave of absence.

The next week was absolute hell. The herbs and vegetables that the holistic doctor gave me seemed to be making my condition worse. I was constantly going to the bathroom and bleeding bright red blood. Another call to my G.I. and I was told by his secretary that he was still on vacation and I should just take more Imodium. I told her that I needed help now or would end up in the hospital. She said she would tell him when he got back. Nice! I was stranded with no place to turn and a few days later I was not able to walk on my own and had to go to the ER. My wife practically carried me in.

After some initial blood work, a CAT scan and stool testing I was admitted to the intensive care unit with severe dehydration and anemia but the doctors still didn't know or tell me what was causing this. The pain meds they gave me helped a little but I was still having urgent diarrhea and had to keep getting up from my hospital bed, dragging the IV unit with me to the bathroom. It was impossible to get any rest in the hospital. I spent 5 days there. The meds they gave me seemed to be calming my guts down some. I was on prednisone and Cipro along with a few other pills that I don't remember. I was released to go home but still in great pain. The diarrhea slowed down some and with the pain meds I could sleep a little. I was glad to get out of the hospital but the severe damage to my intestines would take more than 6 months to heal.

At this point I had to go on Workman's Compensation as I still could not return to work. At 60% of my wages it wouldn't be long until we were so behind in our finances that we would be in a hopeless situation. I had to get back to work ASAP! After a month at home I decided to press my family doctor into releasing me to return to work. She did so reluctantly and I went back thinking this was all behind me now.

I tapered off of the prednisone over the next few months and seemed to be gaining my health back very slowly. I kept thinking that my G.I. was wrong and that I was better now. I was so wrong. Slowly my diarrhea came back and the bleeding started up again. This time I was determined to search the internet for a cause and cure. I knew there had to be answers out there and I would find them. I was not going to let this disease ruin my life!

The Specific Carbohydrate Diet - SCD

As I searched and searched online I kept running into so called cures. All I had to do was send $49.95, or $79.95, or $159.95, and I would be sent the information and/or supplements that were 'guaranteed' to cure me of this disease. The sites had many, many, reviews and they were all extremely positive. Of course I was also very suspicious of these cures. It took a long time, actually several months, before I finally stumbled onto Elaine Gottschall's website Breaking the Vicious Cycle (www.breakingtheviciouscycle.info.) After reading through this site and seeing that they were giving information away for free, I was impressed. I bought the book at Barnes and Noble and began the Specific Carbohydrate Diet (SCD) the next week.

I was absolutely amazed at the results and didn't have a bowel movement for over a week! I was afraid that I was getting blocked up inside even though I had no discomfort. It was a relief to not go for a while. Finally I had a bowel movement and it was not the bloody diarrhea that I was having before. The pain and cramping were subsiding. The diet was fixing me! I steadily improved and quit taking Asacol. I was seeing a new G.I. doctor at the time and he asked me every time I saw him 'how many times per day did you have a BM when you were in high school?' Jesus Christ! That was over 30 years ago! Was it really pertinent? After several visits with him I told him that I quit taking Asacol. He got mad and said that I didn't trust him. I told him that I trusted how I felt and that the Asacol wasn't helping me and that I thought that it was actually hurting me. He threw my chart down on the counter and said fine, call me when you have another flare because you will! I called him alright! Every name in the book! What a jerk! I got my medical history from him a week later and never went back. (Dr. Kiel passed away 8/20/13 due to an accident).

I was convinced that all I needed at this point was the diet. I didn't mind cooking and I didn't care about all the 'illegal foods'. All I cared about was that I was feeling better and could function again. I gained some weight back and was now feeling pretty good. Before this all started I weighed 210 lbs. and I had lost 30 lbs. from the first flare. I was around 180 at this point and felt that it was close to my ideal weight. I had lost a lot of muscle mass too and had to buy new clothes that fit. I went from a 36 waist to a 32! All my shirts were like tents on me. I was following the diet strictly. If I was unsure about anything I did not eat it. I made my own meals, dressings, ketchup, and yogurt. I could eat as much as I wanted and learned how to cook. I bought some really high end knives and learned how to use them. It was fun and I was happy. Feeling much better and hopeful.

I found a new G.I. doctor through my family doctor. He worked for Bayfront Digestive Diseases on State Street almost directly across the street from Hamot Hospital where I had been admitted to the emergency room in 2007. Bayfront Digestive is part of the UPMC health care system and affiliated with Hamot. I found him pleasant but he was unconvinced that diet had anything to do with this disease. I consider it a condition and not a disease. I brought a copy of Breaking the Vicious Cycle with me to show him but he had no interest in it. He wanted to do another colonoscopy but I was terrified of the prep since my first experience was so bad. I sucked it up and agreed to go through with it again because I wanted to show him that the diet had cured me. This time the prep wasn't too bad but the results of the scope were less than I had expected. He said the disease had progressed and that I still had inflammation. In his opinion it was worse than the first colonoscopy. How could that be? I was feeling better. He wanted to put me on Remicade. Doctors must hate the internet! I Googled the side effects and was terrified! No way was I going on that! I had a chest X-ray and test for Tuberculosis and it came back negative, but that scared me. Could Remicade really cause a dormant bacterium to come to life? Sure seemed like it to me. He agreed to allow me to continue on the diet. This doctor was pretty easy going and more than willing to allow me to make my own health decisions. He did warn me of the chance of cancer if left untreated and I understood the risks. I just did not want any immunosuppressant drugs. I felt like I had not explored all of the options yet and that the diet had helped. I still believed that there had to be another answer, another option.

After several years on the SCD I was starting to think I was really cured even though the colonoscopy had shown otherwise. This was October, 2011. I decided to take a chance and eat something that was not allowed on the diet. I had a piece of fresh Italian bread with butter and it was delicious! After a week with no reaction I was happy to try another piece. Another week went by and I was ready to try some breaded chicken Parmesan at a local restaurant. Once again a week passed and no problem. I then tried the lasagna which I knew had a slight amount of sugar in the tomato sauce. A week passed and I was sure I was cured. After a night out we stopped at Taco Bell and I bought 2 regular tacos and ate them both. Man I missed the junk! Still no reaction! Halloween was here and my son in law made some caramel filled dark chocolate candies. I had a couple and they were so good! I had a couple more the next day and that was a big mistake. A few days later I began to notice something weird happening. Oh no! What was going on? I immediately went back on the intro diet but I was going downhill fast. The diarrhea was back and I was noticing blood already! What the hell? I began 40mg of prednisone but to no avail. A couple weeks passed and I was back in the hospital again worse off than I was the first time. I dropped all the weight I had gained and was tipping the scales at around 150. I could not believe it! All the progress I had made was gone and I was back at the beginning. Dammit! The pain this time was excruciating. I felt like I was being torn up from the inside. The sugar was like a nuclear explosion in my gut and there was nothing I could do but suffer through it. I spent another 5 days in intensive care and my doctor didn't come to see me one time. I understand that he was busy but I was there 5 days and his office was kitty-corner to the hospital. He sent a few other doctors to see me but it just made me feel like he didn't really care since he couldn't take 1/2 hour out of his day to visit me. Maybe it was because I refused the drugs and helping him to make his drug quota. I know that seems harsh but money does come into play here. Don't kid yourself.

After getting out of the hospital and again using all my vacation time to recuperate I was forced to return to work too soon. I looked like a holocaust victim! My eyes were sunken and dark, my energy level was so low that I had to be careful about moving too fast and bringing on a dizzy spell, my guts ached and I wasn't sleeping well and yet I had to work or lose everything. I was on prednisone and needed to taper off. My doctor was once again pushing the immunosuppressant drugs. I asked him to give me time to let the diet work again and he reluctantly agreed. Every time I would get down below 5mg/day of prednisone I would begin to have diarrhea and bleeding. The diet wasn't working the same way it had at the beginning. I did the intro diet 3 times and it didn't seem to help. Finally I bought an E book called Surviving to Thriving written by Jordan Reasoner and Steve Wright (www.scdlifestyle.com). In this book were stages of how you should progress on the SCD diet. I followed the stages and was able to wean off of prednisone this time without the problems starting back up. This was a relief and I thought I was finally back on track.

Fecal Transplant?

I was wrong again. Through the rest of 2012 and into 2013 I got progressively worse. The diarrhea continued and I was forced to wear adult diapers. The bleeding had come back and even though I was not in a terrible flare I was making many trips to the bathroom. I was always worried about having an accident. Introducing Tenesmus! The feeling that you have to have a BM but when you try nothing happens. You leave the bathroom but feel you have to go again but once more nothing. This should be renamed torturenesmus. You try to ignore it but then have an accident. So many hours spent on the toilet! My wife waiting and waiting for me to come out of the bathroom. Pure torture!

I tried to add some supplements to my diet because I had been feeling so weak. The supplements - multi vitamin, vitamin B and calcium caused me more problems so I immediately stopped taking them. I tried a probiotic called Critical Care by Renew Life and L-

Glutamine and they seemed to help for a little while but I was still having problems. My situation was getting so desperate that I decided I needed to find a new doctor. I wanted a GI who was unaffiliated with the local hospitals. I found Dr. Brian Bansidhar. He was young and very intelligent. I was hoping he could help me. I had one appointment with him and he stressed how serious this disease (condition) was if left untreated. He was also very concerned with my family's' history of bowel problems and cancer. Once again he did not believe that diet affected bowel function. I brought up the subject of fecal microbiota transplants (FMT) but he said that there was not enough proof through clinical trials to show that it worked for people with UC. I agreed to have a colonoscopy with biopsies taken every 10cm throughout the entire colon. This was performed on Monday and I waited nervously for the test results. They told me that if I didn't hear from them in the next week that the biopsies for cancer were negative. It's hell waiting for a call that would change my life again forever. They should let you know that you are all clear as soon as they have the test results. It's a poor policy and added to my stress.

The first time I read about fecal transplant therapy I nearly vomited. I had to stop reading because I was so grossed out. I didn't understand that there was a procedure to follow. I imagined the worst and it was unthinkable. I slowly got used to the idea and decided to give it another chance. I bought an e-book called Fecal transplant Cures Ulcerative Colitis by Michael Hurst (www.fecaltransplant.org). He suffered from UC for 12 years and was now cured! In his book he outlined the steps that he took to do home fecal transplants to cure his condition. I was convinced that this was the answer. It made perfect sense that the bacteria was out of balance in my gut and needed to be brought back by infusing fecal matter from a healthy donor. The day after my colonoscopy I began to take 60mg of prednisone without the doctors' knowledge to calm the inflammation in preparation for the FMT that I planned to do as soon as healing allowed. When I saw my G.I. again I planned to convince him to partner with me in this. I needed him to supply prescriptions for prednisone, antibiotics and hopefully a sedative so I could follow Michaels' protocol and cure myself. I didn't think he would go along with it but I had nothing to lose and he had no answers or cure. He wouldn't take responsibility if I had a negative reaction from Imuran or Remicade would he? No, so there should not be a problem. I thought that together we could prove that this is curable.

U.C. Is A Bitch

At this point I would like to step back a bit and tell you a little about how U.C. has changed my life.

Before U.C., I was healthy and active. I have always had alot of energy and with the exception of heartburn had no digestive issues. I took Tums for this and eventually started taking Prevacid once a day. I was happy to not have any heartburn anymore after suffering from it from a very early age. I am suspicious of the Proton pump inhibitor drugs (Zantac, Prilosec) now and wonder if they too were somewhat responsible for my getting U.C. These drugs inhibit the formation of stomach acid allowing undigested food to move through the system where bacteria can feed on it in the colon. Not an ideal situation to say the least!

I went from a busy carefree lifestyle to cooking all my meals, checking all labels and avoiding illegal foods, not eating out, no alcohol, loss of energy, and constant fear of being in public without a bathroom nearby or worse yet it being occupied. Our conversations at home revolved around shit! All we talked about was shit! We were talking shit every day, everywhere we went, no matter what we did or how we tried to avoid it the subject would eventually come up. We made jokes about pooping and laughed and cried about it. We were angry at the doctors and at a medical system that didn't care about finding a cure for U.C. The constant push to take Immunosuppressant drugs like Remicade, Imuran, and Humira pissed me off. Doctors do not have incentive to cure people. A new cure will be debated and contested for years. It invites trouble so they simply give in and give up. I know this is a difficult condition to cure and I know that everyone's system is unique but medication is not the answer. I cannot believe how many times I have heard a doctor say that diet has nothing to do with bowel problems. Really? Whatever happened to you are what you eat?

My musical career was on hold, my body ached from malnutrition and I felt like arthritis was affecting my joints. I got mad at myself when I had an accident or we had to change plans because of U.C. There were times when I was feeling good that we decided to go out but as I was on the way had an accident and we had to drive home. This was all so depressing and at times I felt that I wasn't a man at all anymore. I was a shell. I shrank! I was just a little fellow now. I used to be strong and muscular but now I was bony and skinny. I hated it! This was no way to live and I got tired of my life being about shit. There was nowhere to turn and nothing to do so I just learned to take it one day at a time. What else could I do? At least I was still alive. Not much of a life though, compared to how I used to live. It just sucked!

Preparing For FMT

Twelve days since the colonoscopy and the doctors' office hadn't called so I was fairly confident that no cancer was found. I was on prednisone 60mg/day since and had seen remarkable improvement. Not running to the toilet 20 times a day, less accidents, joint pain gone, muscles and tendons loosening up, I even started exercising again! There were some side effects. I would wake up about an hour after falling asleep every night and then every hour after that to pee. I started taking a teaspoon of cannabis leaf and some valerian root to help me sleep. My wife said I seemed grouchy. I felt irritable. My face was rounded out a little. I didn't have moon face (a common side effect from prednisone) yet though. I thought I actually looked better. My cheeks weren't so sunk in. I knew that I couldn't stay on prednisone forever but it sure was a nice break from the flare I was experiencing. I was not bleeding at all. I felt almost normal!

Monday was D day! I would be seeing my G.I. doctor at 2:30 and hopefully would be able to convince him to partner with me in my plan for home fecal transplant therapy. I had been gearing up for this for a few weeks. I bought protein powder (Warrior Force), Vitamin B-12 injections, an iron supplement, L-Glutamine, and even a small dorm sized refrigerator because my wife would not allow me to store poop in the kitchen refrigerator. I probably had around $400 invested. I truly believed that this would work and I was using Michael Hurst's book for guidance. I was planning on 10 days of fecal transplants right before bed. I needed more prednisone, Vancomycin or Cipro, and Bupropion or Silenor from the Doctor. Even if he didn't want to help me I would buy the prednisone online and continue on it until the therapy was complete. I was moving forward with this with him or without him. I planned on weaning off the prednisone after the transplants and hoped that the new bacteria would colonize my system and I would be cured!

I met with my doctor and it went really well. I was upfront about the prednisone even though I was a bit worried that he would be mad at me for self-medicating. He said that he understood that I was in need of something and would have started me on 40mg/day but that 60 was ok if that's what worked for me in the past. That was a relief! I really wanted to work with him and I wanted him on my team.

He told me that all the biopsies came back negative for cancer but made sure I knew that that didn't mean I absolutely didn't have it. They can't biopsy the entire colon so there is a possibility that it can be missed. Even with that I was very relieved. Next we talked about the meds he wanted to use to get me into remission. I was agreeable to Lialda and a slow taper off of prednisone over the next 6 weeks but if I started to have problems again I would up my prednisone because I couldn't go back to bleeding and constant diarrhea. No way! He explained that Liada (Mesalamine) would not get a person out of a flare but could soothe the colon after the prednisone did its work of reducing the inflammation. No other doctor had ever explained this to me and previously I had thought that Mesalamine would work to stop a flare. That was good info. From our first meeting Dr. Bansidhar got the distinct impression that I was totally against any meds. I told him that this was not so and that I was willing to work with him if he would work with me. He assured me that every decision was mine and that his job was to find the best possible solution for me. I appreciated that and told him so.

Now was the time for me to bring up the subject of home fecal transplants again! I brought Dr. Borodys' study (an Australian doctor who has had success in clinical trials treating c. difficile using FMT) and several other papers showing that there was a possibility that the therapy worked. I also brought a condensed version of Michael Hurst's story about how he cured himself. My doctor seemed very interested! He again said that he didn't know everything and that he was interested in this. I explained that I wanted to use my wife as a donor and that I would be doing this at home. I also told him I wanted his help in obtaining Vancomycin and other drugs to make sure I did it right. He said he would read over the info I gave him and consult with some colleagues about it. His advice was to wait until I got the inflammation under control before I started FMT. I agreed and told him it meant a lot to me that he was open to this. He seemed genuinely excited and I truly believed he would help me. I was excited as I left his office and even though I needed to wait a little longer before I started the FMTs I thought the meeting was a success and that I was on the right path. I made an appointment to see him again in 6 weeks. At that time I would hopefully be off the prednisone and healing. That would be the beginning of October and I could then start the therapy.

I went off of the SCD over the weekend starting slowly with some potatoes one day and some bread the next. I had pasta on Sunday and didn't notice any ill effects. It was such a joy to eat like that again and the food made me feel good. We were able to go to a restaurant that we hadn't been to in years and my wife enjoyed a meal that she missed a lot. The diet helped me when nothing else would (before I knew about prednisone) but it didn't cure me. It just put the inflammation down to a tolerable level. I knew bacterial imbalance was the key here. I got involved in the Human Food Project (http://humanfoodproject.com/americangut/) and was looking forward to seeing the difference between my gut bacteria and my wife's. We both sent fecal samples using a kit that they provided. We had to document our meds and food habits for a week. It was cumbersome but I needed to know what was lurking in my gut. I will speak more about this report later in the book.

I hated being sick! It consumed my life for 7 years! I used to be a drummer and I didn't even have a drum set anymore! I used to play guitar. I didn't even have a guitar now! I was learning to play the blues harp and that was getting me through. I had the blues! The poopin' too much blues! It was not fun thinking about U.C. all the time and I was definitely worried about coming off prednisone. I felt really great but I had felt this before. As soon as I dropped the steroid I would start the downward spiral again. I didn't want this to happen. My doctor wanted me to cut the prednisone dosage to 30mg/day for the next week and this scared me. I quit the SCD and had no problems with bread, potatoes, pasta or moms fresh homemade peach pie! She was so happy watching me eat it and I really enjoyed it a lot. I can't tell you how good food tastes when you haven't had it for years! It's absolutely amazing!

Here was my dilemma. I wanted to start the home fecal transplants as soon as possible. It felt like the inflammation had subsided and I was not going to the bathroom as much. I was not bleeding but my stools were still not formed. I told my doctor I would wait until I was off the prednisone and in remission before I started the home therapy. He thought that Lialda might get me to stay in remission as I weaned off the prednisone. I was highly doubtful. I was also thinking that I might be playing with fire by coming off the SCD right now. I knew it was only because of the prednisone that I could eat non-SCD foods. I wanted to start the fecal transplants now! I was considering ordering Cipro and Bupropion from an online Canadian pharmacy and moving forward with this the next week. It's so weird how the mind is affected by bowel conditions. I like to think of myself as a logical and intelligent person but this sickness messes with your brain. I had difficulty making decisions and remembering things. I also felt desperate to get well and I couldn't go through another extreme flare. I didn't want to end up in the hospital again and I didn't want to have my colon removed. I was just so sick and tired of being sick and tired! I wanted to be normal again!

Tuesday morning after the Labor Day holiday I was improving even though I was off the diet. I was eating anything I wanted. I even had ice cream! My stools had gotten progressively harder and because I was still a bit sore I started vitamin E enemas before bed. This brought some relief from the pain while going and the little bit of bleeding I was seeing because of the hard poop had stopped. I had great amounts of energy and felt like my old self. I was at about 80%. I could ride my bike again but I would get tired quickly. I remember when I could ride and ride and ride without feeling the burn in my thighs. I wanted that feeling back! Soon! So here's what I started doing: 2 heaping tbls. Ultimate Warrior Food (chocolate), 1 tsp L-Glutamine (fermented), 1 cup blueberries, or 1 peach, 2 tbls. of honey, 2 tbls. fish oil in a shake each morning for an extreme protein boost, Vitamin B-12 shots (1000mcg-musclular) for 7 days, and then every other day for 7 more injections, 25mg Gentle iron (Solgar Iron Bisglycinate) 2x daily, Freeda calcium (5x), multivitamin (3x), ultimate b (1x) Ultimate Flora Critical Care 50 Billion Probiotic (1x), prednisone 60mg daily, Protonix 30mg - not liking this, Lialda (2x), Valerian root (4x at bedtime), and a vitamin E (D-tocopherol 10x 1000 mg) enema at bedtime

I was off the SCD and eating what I wanted, still eating healthy and only having really bad foods occasionally (cake, ice cream, sweet drinks -no pop).

A Note on the SCD

I want to bring something up that I have experienced that might be somewhat controversial. I don't want to be a downer about the Specific Carbohydrate Diet or discourage anyone from trying it or depending on it. I did for years. The diet calmed my symptoms and allowed me to function without medicine. Here's the problem: Even though I was doing better the inflammation was still there just under the surface. I wasn't really getting better. I was maintaining. How do I know this? Just a week after going off the diet I was in a full blown flare! It didn't take weeks or months, it happened almost immediately. I had a colonoscopy and was told that I was worse than I was 2 years before when I had started the diet. After being on the diet again since my last flare in 2011 my colonoscopy showed the same thing. "Inflamed from stem to stern" is how my doctor put it. He warned me very sternly about letting this inflammation continue. That is why I have decided to stay on prednisone and am moving forward with the FMT. My main point is that even though you might feel that the diet is working and that you are getting better, the inflammation might still be there. It's just not so bad that you are being bothered by it. You cannot let this linger. Cancer is the main threat if you do. Make sure you are getting the inflammation under control. Get a colonoscopy to be sure. That's all I have to say on this for now. I hope everyone can be cured of this terrible condition someday.

Prednisone Taper

Now it was time to begin a taper off of the prednisone. My doctor wanted me to go to 30mg/day but I wanted to stay at 60mg because of all the non SCD food I was eating. I ordered Cipro and Wellbutrin from a Canadian pharmacy without a prescription. The next step would be 5 days of Cipro to weaken the hold that any bad bacteria had in my gut followed by a 10 day regimen of evening fecal transplants while taking the Wellbutrin (Bupropion) to calm my system down while continuing the slow prednisone taper down to zero. I hadn't had any urgency lately so I was thinking my system was ready. I was very excited to be doing this and extremely hopeful that it would be the answer to my hope for a cure.

I decided to give in and lower my prednisone dose to 30mg/day per my doctors' insistence. That night was bad. I started having diarrhea and urgency again and that scared me. I immediately went back to 60mg/day and called the doctor. He was adamant that I stay at

30mg and said that it was probably just a coincidence that I started having problems right after cutting the dose. I wasn't convinced and since I had a wedding to go to on Saturday I told him I was going to stay at 60 until Sunday and then cut it to 30 and see how it goes. I felt better the rest of the week and had a nice time at the wedding without any problems. On Sunday I did as I said and cut the dose to 30. I felt ok Sunday but Monday started going more often and my butt started getting extremely sore. My stools were slightly formed now and somewhat hard making it painful to go, especially 5-6 times a day. I had been eating a lot more than usual. I was so damned hungry all the time! I believe this was from a combination of the prednisone and also my body demanding nourishment. I did gain a few pounds and was up to 174 lbs. as of that morning. I had 5 bowel movements the previous night and 3 in the morning and they were very painful and urgent at times. I didn't know how he could say that the prednisone had the same effect at 30 as it did at 60. He told me that the amount shouldn't matter at this time. It sure seemed to matter to my guts! I was going a couple times a day and suddenly I was going a lot more. I knew I had to cut the prednisone but maybe at a slower rate. I needed to stay healed to do the fecal transplants. I was still waiting for my meds from the Canadian Pharmacy. I hoped they would come soon but I was too sore to do the therapy at this time anyway.

I was continuing to build up my albumen levels with the protein powder and giving myself the vitamin B-12 shots every other day. I stopped the vitamin E enemas because they didn't seem to be helping anymore. I read that coconut oil could be very soothing so I thought I might try that instead. I was not feeling well and had noticed a lot of muscle cramping lately. Not sure what that was from. Probably malnourishment. My hands were getting cramped up just from holding my steering wheel. Very strange. I felt depressed too. Having accidents again made me feel really bad. I was trying to keep my spirits up and was still hopeful that the fecal transplant therapy would cure me. The waiting was killing me though. My doctor was very stingy with the prednisone and my prescription ran out because I stayed at 60mg. for an extra week. I was hoping he would re-fill it for me since I only had a couple days worth left. I knew I would also be buying that from the Canadian Pharmacy soon. It was so expensive though. I payed around $7 for 50 -

10mg pills through my insurance but the Canadian Pharmacy charged around $50. I would have to do it, I had no other choice.

I was still off the SCD and enjoying eating what I wanted. I didn't have any reaction to the foods I was eating. I had pasta for dinner and it was great. I also had a sub from my favorite lunch spot, Marias. They make a killer meatball sub and I got banana peppers, mushrooms and cheese on it. It was great! I went to McDonalds drive thru and ordered a Big Mac. When she said it would be $4.59 I said what??? $4.59 for a Big Mac??? Forget it and I drove away. That was probably for the best. That food is so bad for you. (I really wanted one though hee hee hee!)

I called the pharmacy to see if Dr. Bansidhar had refilled my prednisone prescription but they told me they had not heard from him since they called on Monday. I called him again and told his assistant that I was down to 6 - 10mg pills and would need more soon. She called back and told me they needed me to stay with his taper program which is 30 this week, 15 next week, 10 the week after, 5 the next and 5 every other day for one more week and then stop. I knew he was going to add up exactly how many pills I needed because he didn't want me to have any leftover. I decided to buy from the Canadian Pharmacy. I ordered from here www.thecanadianhealthcaremall.com. I placed the order and got my pills in less than 3 weeks.

I was still having trouble with anal soreness. I wasn't going as much but it was excruciatingly painful when I did. My guts were healing from all the supplements, vitamin B-12 and protein meal replacement shakes. I was not bleeding at all and that was great! I asked Dr. Bansidhars' assistant about the soreness which was just at the end of my rectum and the inside of my cheeks. She said he suggested an ointment called Calmoseptine. I bought some at Walgreens for $5.99 and tried it that night. It did not help at all. The only thing that helped was rinsing with a warm spray in the tub after going and applying Vaseline after I dried. I couldn't do that at work though so I would just wet some TP and dab. I tried some Bacitracin in a tube and that helped. It seemed like my stools were made of pure acid!

Dr. Bansidhar insisted that I go on Protonix to make sure I didn't get a stomach ulcer from the high dose of prednisone. I had been on Protonix before as well as other Proton pump inhibitors and they worked well for me. No heartburn at all. Having anal pain is enough! Flaring and having extremely painful heartburn at the same time is no fun at all. That is why I agreed to take it again. I am not sure how good it is for me and I am suspicious that that is why my stools were so acidic. I needed to do something to make my stools less painful. I knew that coming off the SCD may have been responsible for this but after eating anything I wanted I didn't want to go back. I didn't know if I could. The thought just bummed me out so bad. I was not reacting to anything. I just had to get healed up to do the FMT. I would go back on the diet if this didn't clear up in the next few days. Pooping was so painful that I dreaded going. I could hardly walk after, it was awful. I was glad I had an elevated desk at work that allowed me to stand and work. I could not sit for more than a few minutes.

Another thing I want to mention is that I had been taking 1 tsp. of dried cannabis leaf and Valerian root (530 mg x 4) before bed. That really helped me sleep. Sleep is very important. I know medicinal cannabis is illegal and if the government wants to bust me then I say come get me. I am trying to be as honest and helpful as I can. That is why I am telling you everything. I want you to know my experience and I am hoping it will help you or your loved one. No one should suffer like this!

My doctor had me lower the dose of prednisone to 30mg/day starting on a Sunday. I did ok and really didn't have any problems other than the ones I have been having with the soreness and acidic stools. I had been having 8-10 BMs a day and some gas and urgency. They were very painful and it felt like I was crapping razor blades. A week later he had me lower the dose by 1/2 again to 15 mg/day. I did ok on Sunday but had a rough night sleeping Sunday night and woke with a headache and slight fever (101.6°) Monday morning. It was hell going to work with chills and a headache but I made it through the day.

That night I was freezing and had a hard time sleeping. I had 3 BMs during the night and 3 more in the morning. I got to work ok but as soon as I got there I had to run to the bathroom. I nearly had an accident. My temp that morning was 99.6° and I woke with a headache and tightness in my lungs. Reading online, these symptoms are indicative of a too fast taper off prednisone. Dr. Bansidhar gave me a prescription for 28-10mg pills. That wasn't much. He wanted to force me off the prednisone ASAP. After my colonoscopy I put myself on 60mg/day. I was honest with him about that and he asked me where I got the prednisone. I told him I had it leftover. Apparently he didn't like that and was making sure I didn't have any leftover this time.

I had to follow his taper schedule because I was sure he would not prescribe any more. I was also reading that you should not take antibiotics while tapering off prednisone. I planned on staying at 10 while doing the home FMT. I had the Cipro and Welllbutrin but could not proceed with the therapy until I got the soreness under control.

Not sure what was causing the acidic stools but I quit all supplements in hopes that would help. I was still taking the meal replacement shakes and had added a tablespoon of fish oil. I also made the shake with an Avocado. I was hoping the oils in the Avocado might offer some relief. Maybe this would help. If not I would discontinue the Warrior Food next. If that didn't make a difference I would stop the Protonix. It was so painful having a BM that I would nearly pass out. I had to use wet toilet paper to wipe and was also using Bacitracin at night. I tried the Calmoseptine again and it seemed to soothe. I also tried A & D ointment from Walgreens, it was very soothing and I highly recommend it.

Should I call Dr. Bansidhar today and let him know what is happening? Will he care? Will he do anything to help me? Somehow I didn't think so. Finding a new doctor is such a pain in the ass. It's a crapshoot! I know. That doesn't seem very funny. I tried to see the humor in that but I was feeling so shitty. I was trying to stay positive but feeling depressed again. I was so cold and tired and my body and skin ached. I had been getting really annoying muscle cramps in my hands and the front of my lower legs. Sitting on the toilet and having a painful BM is just so much fun but when your legs are cramping at the same time. It's just unbelievable. How much pain could a person endure? I was finding that amount to be a lot. More than I ever thought.

Now it was a week since I talked to my doctor and he hadn't called me back. I stayed on 20mg/day prednisone all last week and cut to 17 on Sunday. I was feeling good and the burning and soreness were practically gone now. I didn't want to start the fecal transplants that week because we were planning a long weekend trip to see a band so I would start the antibiotic the following Monday and start the FMT the following week. I planned to stay at 10mg/day of prednisone throughout the FMT and then after 10 days of that wean slowly and see how it went. I ordered 180 - 10mg pills of Prednisolone from the Canadian health & Care Mall http://thecanadianhealthcaremall.com/ for $75. Now I could taper at my own pace.

I was a bit upset with my doctor for not staying in communication with me. I thought that he was probably mad that I was not following his prednisone taper schedule. I found this online http://mpkb.org/home/othertreatments/corticosteroids/weaningoffsteroids and it made much more sense than his fast tapering schedule. We are individuals and know how we feel. Doctors need to be aware of that and treat us accordingly. I stopped the protein meal replacement shakes in the morning for a couple days to see if that was why I was getting such bad cramping. I was still experiencing some hand cramping and I was not sure if that was what was causing it or not. The only things I was taking now were Lialda 1.2gm 2x daily, Protonix 1x daily, 17 1/2mg prednisone, and B-12 injections 2X/week.

I was feeling better but still having too many BMs. I was going 6-8 times a day but they were nearly formed and the diarrhea had subsided. No blood or mucus either. I was still having some urgency but some of that was just the panic response I had learned from years of having this condition. I was trying to get better control of my emotions when faced with an attack. I thought if I just relaxed and calmed myself I could avoid accidents. The Zen of pooping! Ha ha! Maybe I'll write a book!

We had a nice 4 day weekend in Jim Thorpe.PA. What beautiful scenery as it was the peak of the leaf season. I was feeling good and had lowered my prednisone to 15mg/day without any problems. I started on Cypro 500mg/day on Monday. I planned to take that for 7 days and then start the home fecal transplants. I was a bit nervous about taking an antibiotic. I was hoping it wouldn't affect my system negatively and give me diarrhea. That would be devastating at this point. I was relatively healed up and ready to do the FMT. It had been a long road getting here and I would hate anything to ruin it now. My wife was having loose stools at the time so I spoke to my daughter and granddaughter about using them as donors. I wanted to do everything I could to make sure this worked. Good donations were paramount! They agreed after the initial shock. I explained that they might just be saving my life! It was weird having that conversation. My granddaughter Mina kept breaking out laughing! It was a strange thing to ask for sure!

I cancelled my appointment with Dr. Bansidhar and re-scheduled for the following week. They were very understanding about that. It would be interesting to see his reaction when I told him I was still at 12.5 mg prednisone and planned on staying at 10 until I completed the FMT. Now that I could get prednisone online I could taper at my own pace.

I was feeling very good and gained some weight. I was at 179 lbs. now! Eating more carbs really helped me gain. I actually thought about not doing the fecal transplant but I knew that the condition still existed and I needed to move forward with this to cure myself. Next Tuesday would be D day for no more D! I was excited to get it done and still very hopeful that I would be cured. I would be taking Wellbutrin also and planned on at least 10 days of FMT. I was hoping for a UC free life!

In the next section I explain the procedure for fecal transplantation and explain the details. It gets quite graphic so be forewarned.

I Start FMT

I did the first home fecal transplant before bed Tuesday night. The weeks of preparation really paid off as I was feeling very good. I was down to 12mg/day prednisone and not experiencing any signs of flaring. My colon felt healed and I was having near solid stools. I was still going too often though, averaging 8-10 BMs/day. I still had urgency and also had a couple accidents over the previous 2 weeks. For seven days I took 500mg of Cipro to weaken the bacteria in my system. Along with the prednisone I was also taking 2 Lialda pills per day and one Protonix.

The one problem I was having was getting a fresh donation. My wife left one for me that she made in the morning before work and it sat in the refrigerator from 6:00 am until 9:45 pm when I used it. I asked my daughters to help me also and was hoping for some evening donations. Even though it sat in the fridge all day I was still hoping to benefit from it. I took 2 Imodium, 2 Valerian root caps, 1 tsp. cannabis leaf, and

300 mg Wellbutrin about an hour before the transplant. I mixed the stool with warm distilled water (not saline) in a blender on low for about 20 seconds and then strained it into a large measuring cup using a wire mesh strainer. I stirred in the psyllium fiber powder with a plastic spoon. At this point I got the bright idea to take all my implements to the basement so I could rinse everything as I did not want to go down 2 flights of stairs after doing the transplant. I thought that was brilliant until I got back upstairs and found that the psyllium fiber had thickened the solution to the point that I could not suck it up into the turkey baster. After that I added the fiber right before I was ready to use the solution. I had to add water to thin it out but the bulb on the turkey baster still gave me trouble. It was way too soft and when I tried and squeeze the solution out and into me it leaked air so I had to hold it around the collar with one hand to seal it and squeeze the bulb with the other. That was very awkward but I got the job done. I needed a better baster! I was able to insert 3 basterfulls. I rolled onto my left side for a couple minutes and then on my right side, upside down bicycle position for a bit and then on my back. I rinsed the container and baster in the upstairs sink and disinfected

it and went straight to bed. I was able to keep the solution in all night and didn't have a bowel movement until about 4:30 am. It was near solid too. I felt great the next day and I thought that I could get used to doing this. It's not as bad as I thought it would be and I just kept my nose plugged for the whole thing. I had an appointment to see Dr. Bansidhar that day at 2:30. I was going to tell him what I was doing and hoped he would help. Either way I was keeping him as my GI for now just in case I needed him.

I saw the doctor and got a stern lecture regarding following his directives. He was angry with me for not tapering the prednisone according to his schedule. I told him that as soon as I went from 30mg to 15mg I started to have problems. He said that couldn't happen and that it was just a coincidence. It was also a coincidence that as soon as I started taking 30mg again the problems stopped. I asked him why every doctor has a different tapering schedule. He said that every patient is different and that it has to be done with regards to the other medications the patient is taking and their current condition. He insisted that I do as he says from now on so I lied and agreed. I was staying on my own taper of -2.5mg per week. I really don't like doctors. Dr. Bansidhar is younger than any other G.I. I have seen and I was hoping we could work together but it's his way or the highway. I didn't mention anything about fecal transplants. I gave him some case studies the last time I saw him and he said he would read them. I don't believe he has any interest in curing this condition. I asked about tapering off the Lialda but he said that I would probably be on that for the rest of my life. I had other plans. I sure hoped this FMT worked. I would like to go the rest of my life without ever seeing a doctor again! My father is 84 and swore off doctors when he was 40. I truly believe that many people die because of the years of taking medications that are supposed to help them. I want to say no to their pharmaceuticals.

The next night's donation came from my daughter and it was much fresher. I mixed it with a fresh donation from my wife. The turkey baster was still giving me problems and I wished I would have investigated better solutions for that. I thought about putting a hose clamp on the bulb. That would seal it and stop the air from leaking out. The other problem is that I had to keep the bulb squeezed while pulling the baster out. Otherwise it would suck the solution right back up and out of me. That was a real pain. I wished there was a better way. I put 2 basterfulls in but couldn't hold it. Luckily I had spread some paper towels out under me so it was an easy clean up. I put another basterfull in but once again I couldn't hold it and headed for the toilet. I still had some in there so I cleaned up and went to bed. I slept well and didn't have a BM until I had a cup of coffee in the morning. It was nearly solid. Putting a turkey baster up your butt isn't fun. I wanted to make sure the solution got in as far as possible because if you only get it in the end of the colon it's much harder to hold. I put the baster in about 5 inches. Once I got it lined up correctly it didn't hurt. Getting the correct angle could be tricky but I was getting better at it. I used Vaseline to coat the baster making it easier to slide in. I couldn't wait until this was over but I was committed to doing it and would continue for 10 days. I thought one baster full was enough. Better to do that and keep it in than to try and put more in and lose it. So far I didn't have any negative side effects from this procedure.

Day 9 of my home fecal transplant experiment and things were going well. I bought a new baster at Walmart for $2. It had a black rubber bulb that fit very snugly over the tube. It worked great and I was so glad I bought it. The tube was made of clear, smooth plastic and was a bit narrower than the previous one. It didn't leak air at all. So far I had been able to hold the solution all night every night. I found that if I could have a bowel movement in the evening, preferably right before the transplant, it made it easier to hold. Makes sense since there is room then. I also found that if I pulled the baster out a little while squeezing the bulb it went in much easier. I was getting good at this! Still I didn't want to continue more than 10 days. The whole process took about 40 minutes and I was getting to bed rather late.

I felt good and believed the therapy was working. I had gotten excited about other remedies before and been disappointed so I was trying to not get too excited while maintaining a positive attitude. I believed it would work. I was still on 10mg prednisone so I wouldn't know for another 4 weeks how I would react once I was totally weaned off of that. I thought the Imodium, Wellbutrin, Valerian root, and Cannabis helped to calm my system and helped me to keep the solution in. The fiber I added also thickened it up after I put it in and I believe this is essential. The bacteria can feed on this and it will populate better.

When I started I was having 6-8 bowel movements a day, now I was down to 4-5. That was progress and I also gained more weight. I was 182 lbs. now! Just call me fatty! Hey, hey, hey! I started exercising again and that felt good. I didn't make a follow up appointment with Dr. Bansidhar. He wanted to see me again in April and do another colonoscopy in August. I wasn't sure if I would go back to him or not. I guess I wanted to wait and see how things went. Two more transplants to go! I would be glad when this was over. It wasn't that bad but not that fun either. It goes to show how desperate a person can be to regain their health and get their life back.

I did the 10th infusion. I was worried because I did not have a donation as of 8:00 PM but my wife came through at the last minute. She was so supportive and encouraging through all of this and I really appreciate her. I didn't feel like doing the transplant but forced myself to go through with it. I had a bit of trouble holding it in and lost some but the majority stayed and I was able to sleep through the night with it in once again.

I started feeling a pain under my right jaw on Wednesday night but just attributed it to doing crunches all week on my incline bench. I was only up to 12 reps but I thought that maybe I strained my neck. I woke in the morning to swelling in my neck under my right jaw. This is where the lymph node is and I was very concerned. I read that swollen lymph nodes are the result of a viral or bacterial infection somewhere in the body and that it usually clears up by itself. It was still swollen the next morning but not worse. I had a bad sliver in my finger that got infected and I got that out. I was hoping that was all it was. My gut felt fine and on the way to work I had to go to the bathroom pretty bad. I was able to hold it even though it was difficult. I felt great about that! It gave me even more hope that this was going to work!

Over the next month I would be tapering very slowly off of the prednisone and then after I saw how I was doing I planned to taper off the Lialda. My doctor wanted me to get blood work done again. I wasn't exactly sure what he was looking for but I figured it wouldn't hurt, especially with the swollen gland. I was hoping that cleared up soon.

My only concern through all of the FMT therapy was that on a few days I had to use donations that were in the refrigerator since early morning. That's one thing I had no control over. I had hoped that since I recruited 3 people to be donors I would have at least one fresh donation every day. If this didn't work that would probably the reason. I read that the fecal matter is only viable for around 6 hours if refrigerated. I would do this again if it was necessary but next time would make sure that I only used fresh donations.

I was feeling good except for the pain under my jaw. Still having 5-6 BMs per day. I was hoping that would lessen over the next couple weeks. I was not having any diarrhea, mucus, or bleeding and my gut felt healed.

I had a nice weekend and it was great to not have to do the fecal transplants. I hoped I wouldn't ever have to do them again but if it didn't work this time I would be willing to try again. I was having 5-6 BMs per day and they were soft. I woke up in the morning very depressed and I was not sure why. I took the last of the Wellbutrin before bed and didn't sleep well. I felt down all day. I was very tired when I got home from work and didn't want to do anything. I slept a little better that night but had strange dreams.

I was still feeling a bit low the next morning and I was having some discomfort in my ascending colon. It was a dull ache. My first thoughts were that I was getting inflamed but I was hoping that wasn't happening. Still no diarrhea so that was a good sign. I was at 7.5mg/day of prednisone and hadn't noticed any changes. I was not restricting my diet either. I even had a couple beers over the weekend!

It's weird but I was thinking about having U.C. and something I read. It said 'you do not know failure in life until you crap yourself'. I remember every single accident vividly. I stopped thinking of it as failure. I dreaded it and even though I always had a clean-up kit and spare diaper with me, I still dreaded it. It was an awful feeling and I sometimes thought of UC as a demon, a living thing that just wanted to destroy my life and make me feel bad about myself. As an example, my wife and I went out of town for 4 days. I had no problems at all for the whole time until we got home. I pulled into the driveway, got out of the truck and immediately had to go. Before I could even get the key in the door I had crapped myself! What the hell? There went all my confidence and I felt like the demon U.C. was laughing at me! I tried to not let it get me down but it was difficult. This battle was not only physical but psychological as well. Now even the slightest feeling of having to go started to put me in a panic. I tried to settle myself and use meditation practices to calm down but nothing seemed to stop it. I also felt a dependency on Depends. When I could go a month or so without an accident or a close call I would begin to try and live without them. Someday I knew I would wear regular underwear again! I swore I would defeat the demon!

A week after I finished doing the 10 fecal transplants I was doing well. I lowered my prednisone to 5mg/day without any ill effects. My stools were still soft and I was going 5-6 times per day. I noticed that if I had my afternoon cup of coffee I usually had to go again but if I didn't I wouldn't have another BM for the rest of the day. I stopped getting up in the middle of the night also and was sleeping much better. My swollen gland under my jaw settled down and the pain in my ascending colon was gone. I was eating and drinking anything I wanted which was very enjoyable.

Since I was still on 2 - 1.2 gm Lialda/day and taking prednisone I couldn't know for sure if the fecal transplants had cured me yet. In the past when I was down to 5mg/day of prednisone I would start having problems but I hadn't been on an ASA medication (Lialda) for a long time so that may have been affecting things. I guess I wouldn't know for sure until I was totally off all medication. I was hoping to see more improvement by now, hoping my stools would be more solid and I would be going less. I took a couple Imodium pills one morning and only had one cup of coffee to see if that would help. I went a couple weeks without an accident so I decided to try and go all weekend without adult diapers. That felt great! Sleeping through the night was also wonderful.

I started exercising again. I was doing a light 10-15 min. workout in the morning, including crunches, rowing, pushups, toe touches, and deep knee bends. I gained more weight and was now at 186+. I had alot of shirts that no longer fit and some of my jeans were too tight now so I decided to buy some new clothes to celebrate! Some joy was returning to my life after all these years of suffering.

I was experiencing joint pain and my right shoulder started hurting really bad for no apparent reason. My knees hurt a bit when I walked but nothing like they used to. My left knee was feeling really bad as though it would allow my leg to go forward. Straightening my leg out all the way was painful. I could still feel this but it was much less and I thought that exercise would help. Overall I was at about 90% and had much improved energy. My spirits were up and I was very hopeful. When I thought of the past 7 years I was amazed at what I had been through and how much pain I had endured. The diet was so stifling to our lifestyle. It was so nice to be able to stop and have lunch anywhere we wanted. I had no urgency and had to go badly on the way to work one day but was able to hold it for over 10 minutes! There is life after U.C.!

I was doing pretty good but noticed some changes in the past few days. I was now at 4.5mg/day prednisone and taking 2 - 1.2 gm/day Lialda. I had more gas and some wetness but no blood. That made me anxious. I had some urgency and close calls too. I went alot the following day, 9 times. I even went a couple times before bed and that was unusual. I felt a bit down again and was afraid that I was going to start flaring. I thought I might do more transplants but only fresh and in the evening before bed if possible. I was not ready to give up yet!

I thought about going back on the SCD but really didn't want to. I was trying to eat better during the week but got a little crazy on the weekends. I knew this might have been be foolish. I had two beers and some vodka on Saturday night. We danced and had a good time. I didn't notice any digestive issues Sunday morning but I had a bad headache most of the day. I thought it best stop drinking beer for now and stop mixing alcohols. I had cake and Ice cream on Sunday and didn't have a reaction. I ate at TGIF and didn't even have to go until right before bed and it wasn't an emergency. Many times at restaurants I would get my food and take one bite and have to run to the bathroom only to sit there with nothing happening. I felt bad for my wife who had to eat alone quite often. The sensation is called tenesmus. When your bowel is inflamed you feel like you have to go all the time. It's enough to drive a person crazy! I had been going without adult diapers but I did get nervous so I thought I would stick with them for a little while longer. I hated to depend on them but it's a crutch I was not ready to give up just yet.

I gained another pound and was now at 187+. I was still exercising and increasing my reps. It felt good to have some energy back. I still worried and this condition had me conditioned to worry. I knew it would take years to heal both physically and emotionally. I continued to hope for the best. Maybe a few more transplants were needed. Only time would tell.

I did another transplant. It was difficult and I had to do it 3 times before I was able to hold it in. That was hard! I felt much better later in the week, with much more energy and I started to feel positive about the FMT again. I had tried so many things without success. I didn't want to be let down again. I was cautiously optimistic.

We had a Birthday party for my 10 year old granddaughter on Sunday. I had fun and it was so nice to join in on the snacks, cake and ice cream. I saw a little blood on Monday morning and that really bummed me out. Not dark red but more of a pink color but there was no denying that it was blood. This may have been related to eating so much sugar on Sunday. I didn't have diarrhea but did have some urgency. I saw a flash of a future that included Remicade or Humira or even surgery. Man that was scary! I sure as hell didn't want to go there.

I stopped taking the protein breakfast replacement shakes and lowered my Prednisone to 4mg/day. I was still taking Lialda but wanted to stop taking Protonix soon. I weighed 189+ now!

After seeing the blood on Monday morning I was really depressed. I didn't see any more the rest of the day or the next morning so I was hopeful again. I was having too many bowel movements each day. I went 9 times that day! That was hard on me and even though I was not having diarrhea I had some urgency and had a really close call at work. This shit was nerve racking!

It was nice to go out on Saturday and have a few drinks. I stuck to Tanqueray and tonic and stayed away from the beer. I had a slight headache on Sunday but nothing too bad. I enjoyed seeing some old friends and they all were amazed at how much better I looked. I didn't talk about U.C. but just said thanks. I also didn't talk about my sickness with my family at the Birthday party on Sunday. That was awesome! I realized that I am not one of those people who like the attention that sickness brings (Munchausen syndrome). I wanted to be better and I longed for a day when I wouldn't have to think about U.C. There was a bright, beautiful future for me and I knew it was going to start soon!

Progress Diary

I kept a journal of my progress. It's the best way for you to see how the healing occurred. It took many years to get sick so it would take quite some time to get better.

11/20/2013

After lowering the prednisone dosage below 5mg per day I always seem to have problems. This time was no different. All last week I noticed more mucus and looser BMs. I ate dinner at Bob Evans on Friday evening and had the chicken Alfredo penne pasta. This brought on a bad reaction. I was thinking I was going to end up back in the hospital. That's how bad it was all through the night. On Saturday morning I upped my prednisone. I took 5mg then and 5mg at dinner. My system settled down and I was fine by Saturday evening. I can tell you now that I was really scared as I have spent too many holidays recovering from flares.

I actually started bleeding Friday night and even today noticed some blood. Nothing heavy but undeniably there. I thought I was in remission and healed up inside but this leads me to believe that wasn't true. Does prednisone simply mask the symptoms? That's what my G.I. said. Maybe he is right. I don't really know the best course of action to take now. I can still function with prednisone and I hate the idea of trying something else. I don't want to have my colon removed either. This really sucks!

As you know by now my idea was that after doing a series of fecal transplants I could wean from the meds and be cured of U.C. I believe it takes a long time to get everything back to normal. My tentative plan now is to stay at 10mg Prednisolone until the end of the year and then slowly drop back to 5mg and wean to zero slowly while watching for any problems.

1-6-2014

The New Year is here and I am still doing pretty well. I made it through the holidays without any issues. It is taking much longer than I thought it would but I am beginning to think the fecal transplant worked. I have been off Lialda now for a week without any noticeable changes. I have lowered my prednisone to 7.5 mg per day. I still go too many times a day but I think it's because of the damage to my colon. I won't know for sure until I am totally off the meds. Like I said I am still hoping I am cured.

1-23-2014

I am down to 3mg prednisone per day and am off all other drugs except 1 Protonix per day for heartburn. I have been eating anything I want and gaining weight. I am currently holding steady at 193. I still go to the bathroom a lot but no blood and I am beginning to have more control. This is great! I received my bacterial data back from American Gut a few weeks ago and sure enough it shows that my bacteria is a lot different than the rest of the people who had the test. I will expound on this more later. For now I feel great and am doing well. I am beginning to think that this will be successful after all!

1-28-2014

I have an appointment with Dr. Bansidhar this afternoon but I am going to cancel. I just don't want to see him. I am feeling pretty good and I believe I am on my way to being cured of Ulcerative Colitis. As of Sunday I am on 2mg/day prednisone and 1 Protonix. I started taking 2 Tablespoons of extra virgin olive oil per day also just I because I think it is good for me. I am still making the protein meal replacement shakes with the Warrior Food a couple times a week to keep my Albumen levels up and 1 to 2 vitamin B-12 shots weekly (intramuscular).

I have 8-10 BMs per day and they are small and sometimes formed. I have no gut pain, no gurgling and very little gas. I am eating what I want and weigh 193 lbs. now. I have started taking Epsom salt baths 1-2 times a week to see if I can relieve some of my joint pain. The joint pain is mainly in my knees but I also feel stiffness in my lower back. My wife says maybe that's just because I am getting old. I just laugh at that! I have no bleeding and have not had an accident in well over a month. Last Saturday evening we went to our club to hear some live rock music and do some dancing. I had to take a crap as soon as we got our drinks. I went into the men's room and the toilet was occupied and there is only one stall so I had to wait. I waited over 10 minutes and was very proud that I could hold it that long. I didn't have a diaper on either! We danced and had a great time the rest of the evening!

American Gut Sample Results

Now I would like to go over the results of my American Gut sample. If you haven't heard of this it's a group of scientists that have joined together to study the micro biome (what bacteria we have in our guts). Here's a link if you're interested in learning more about the project www.americangut.org.

My sample shows that the bacteria in my gut are quite different than the majority of other people's samples. I have high levels of Firmicutes, low Proteobacteria, very low Bacteroidetes, and moderately high levels of Actinobacteria. Other samples show some Tenericutes and Cyanobacteria but mine has none. Isn't that interesting? It's no wonder that I have found some balance after doing the fecal transplant. This test proves that my bacteria were out of whack and I am so glad I spent the money to verify that!

I believe the problems I am still having are related to the damage my colon has experienced from the long bouts of diarrhea. I am healing very slowly. I think this is the cure and I will continue to update you on my progress. Please feel free to ask questions and I would highly recommend that you consider FMT if you are suffering from Ulcerative Colitis. The idea that our immune system is malfunctioning is wrong. It is functioning as it should considering the condition of our systems.

Progress Diary Cont.

2/10/2014

Last week I increased my intake of extra virgin olive oil to 2 tablespoons in the morning and 2 in the evening. I noticed that I started having looser stools and Friday it felt like I was pooping acid! I didn't take the Friday evening dose and haven't had any all weekend. I feel much better today. Extra virgin olive oil is hot when you swallow it and for me it was hot coming out too. It may benefit some people but not me.

I quit the prednisone Saturday and cut my Protonix by half. I feel great today and haven't gone more than a few times. I think I may have a donor from outside the family for doing another transplant. I believe I would benefit from that. I plan on doing only one and seeing how it goes. It's been a long time since I was able to get off prednisone and I am happy about that. I am still eating anything I want but being careful to eat mostly healthy. I love pizza and honey mustard wings. I can also have pasta and bread without any reaction.

I am very happy I did the fecal transplant and am still healing. Life is good and I have planned a vacation with my wife in the late spring. I feel like I have my life back!

2/24/2014

I decided to see my GI doctor even though I don't need to. I guess it's like paying a retainer to keep him on. I can take my info from American Gut and show him the disparity of my bacteria. It will be interesting to hear his thoughts on that. My appointment is today at 4:30. I am sure he will not be happy that I quit the Lialda. I hate taking medicines that don't seem to do anything. I think they can cause more problems.

I have been feeling steadily better, especially this weekend. I still have many BMs throughout the day, averaging 8-10. I only went 5-6 times on Saturday and today only 4 so far. That's pretty good for me. As I have stated previously, I have damage to my colon therefore I have to relieve myself often. My stools are still soft but not diarrhea. It's just a matter of time until I am totally healed. I have no gut pain and don't have to run to the BR.

I have been trying to find a donor outside the family but am finding it difficult. I think if I could do another couple transplants I could speed up the process. It takes a long time for the bacteria to stabilize and for the balance to be found. I am on the right track and haven't felt this good in years. I have some joint pain in my knees. This may be something I just have to live with.

I hope you try fecal transplant and it works for you as well as it has for me. Good luck!

3/25/2014

I am still improving. I did another transplant from a male donor outside the family. He was hesitant which can easily be understood but finally saw it as a good thing. I had a hard time doing that one. I tried 3 times before I was able to hold it. I did not think it would be that bad. I think it's because I'm full of shit now. Hahaha! I have gained back almost all of the weight I lost since I first got sick. I was 220 then (slightly overweight) and am now holding steady at 196. I can't say I am totally 100% but I am doing well and able to function again. I believe that the healing just takes a long time.

I saw Dr. Bansidhar last month and he was amazed at how good I looked. He wanted to schedule me for an upper GI but I refused this. I am tired of the tests and his explanation was that he wanted to see if there were any stomach issues because of my heartburn. I have been on Protonix for a few months now but finally quit those cold turkey last Friday. I should not have done that. I should have gone to an H2 blocker and then weaned off of that. I got really bad heartburn Saturday and Sunday. It's called bounce back. The Proton pump inhibitor stops the stomach from making acid and when you take it away the system bounces back and creates much more than needed. I started taking fresh squeezed lemon juice in a glass of warm water in the morning to see if that would help. I also take 1 tsp. of baking soda in a glass of water when the heartburn gets unbearable. I didn't have heartburn very much when the doctor started me on the Protonix. He wanted me to take it because the prednisone is hard on the stomach. I wish I had not started taking it. I do not want to be dependent on any drugs.

I totally believe in the fecal transplant as the cure for Ulcerative Colitis!

4/8/2014

I think I found the cure for my heartburn! After stopping the Protonix I had a couple real bad episodes. I would take baking soda or a Tums at home but when I was away from home I didn't have anything so I drank water to quash the burn. I found that the water helped right after I drank it but the heartburn would come right back and would sometimes get worse. This got me to thinking about water. I started drinking a lot of water nearly 30 years ago with the idea that hydration was imperative. I still think it is but I don't know if everyone needs to drink a lot of it and I actually think it was causing my heartburn! I did an experiment yesterday and drank much less. No heartburn all day. Today I squeezed lemon in my water bottle and have only been sipping on that. Still no heartburn. Is it possible that the water has been diluting my stomach acid causing indigestion? Seems possible. I am going to continue to limit my water intake and not drink at all with meals to see if this is really the answer. I feel pretty confident right now.

I am still feeling pretty good. My stools are not perfect and I am going more than I want to. I am having a lot of gas too. The only way to tell if the FMT therapy is a success is to wait and see. I am doing better than I have in years and am pretty convinced that this is the answer. Getting the gut bacteria balanced may be a lifetime project.

I read an article about Rheumatoid Arthritis patients having increased occurrences of IBS and IBD. The article attributed that to steroids and Nsaids and said to contact your doctor. It also said that not much was known about the causes of these conditions and that they were auto immune diseases. Bullshit! These are conditions caused by prescription drugs or bacterial imbalance and they do not know how to treat them because their drugs are the cause. They are afraid to look at bacterial imbalance because every system is different and they can't figure it out. They want easy answers and so do we. I hope American Gut can find some real answers with their studies. That is the only hope for RA and IBS/IBD patients!

4/21/2014

I went out of town for a couple days for the Easter weekend. I don't know if it was the stress of driving or staying in a motel room, eating differently or what but I did have some urgency and actually had an accident on the way home. I took Imodium last Monday to help me get through a day of meetings at work and it did help as I had no problems but I think I got a little backed up. I always seem to have to pay later when I take Imodium. I am going to avoid it from now on.

I am feeling good even though I did see some trace amount of blood over the weekend. I weigh 193 now and have been holding steady there for the past couple months. I notice a lot of wetness in my BMs lately and some mucus also. I saw white streaks the other day and Googled it. It said it could be the result of the gall bladder not processing fats. I think it was just mucus. I feel better today and had our family's traditional Easter soup yesterday and some cheese cake that my mom makes every year. When I was on SCD I thought that I would never be able to eat these things again so that was a real treat after 6 years!

I started walking again at lunchtime. My knees have felt like they could let my legs collapse and when I tighten my knees up and push my lower leg forward I feel pain. Walking seems to help and my knees feel a little better. I have to be careful. I feel like if I'm not I could fall and pull something and get hurt badly. I never felt this until I got U.C. I tried a rowing machine and I tried deep knee bends which I can do easily but these exercises don't seem to help much. I decided to ease back into exercising this morning with some crunches, pushups, toe touches and stretching. I can't wait to start riding my bicycle again!

5/15/2014

I am continuing to improve. My only problems stem from damage to my colon from the doctors waiting too long to help me. I get very angry when I think about how they put me off and how I may have to suffer for the rest of my life because of it. Even though I am not having diarrhea I still have urgency. When I have to go I have only a few minutes to make it to the restroom. This isn't always convenient and I am having accidents on rare occasions. If the doctors would have put me on prednisone immediately I would have avoided the damage and might be 100% right now. Bastards!

Enough of that. I told you I had started taking walks again and that has been awesome! I dropped 5 lbs. recently and was worried until I realized that it was just because I was getting that mile+ walk every afternoon. My knees still ache and I have alot of stiffness but it seems to be improving. Maybe I will try to find a natural remedy for joint pain. The peppermint tea helps for the heartburn. That has subsided to a manageable level. I have most of my energy back and am once again taking projects on. My most recent venture is learning to play the blues harp and repairing, tuning, and customizing harmonicas. I am in the process of building a harmonica tuner. That's pretty exciting and I feel like my old adventurous, inventive self again. I don't know if I will ever be able to play music for a live audience again because of the bathroom emergencies but maybe someday. I might even talk to my G.I. about surgery to repair the damage. Maybe. Probably not.

6/6/2014

My weight is holding at 193. I wish I could get back to exercising daily. It seems like every time I start I end up with some kind of pain. I did 20 crunches on my incline bench before I went on vacation and ended up with a pinched nerve in my back. It didn't happen right away but lasted all week. It was actually more in my left hip and then moved to include my right hip also. Then I got another pain in my back in the Latissimus dorsi m. muscle that hurt until today. It's still sore but feeling much better now. I won't stop trying to stay in shape. Monday I will start my routine again. The walking has helped my knees even though I feel that collapsing feeling like my knees are going to buckle backwards. I hate that!

Last week I was on vacation. It was great to get some stuff done around the house and to get out of town for a couple days. I drank a couple beers early in the week and then had bad gas the rest of the week. Honestly I don't know if it was the beer. I seem to be cycling. I do well for a day or two and then I do badly for a day or two. I did see a small amount of blood last week. Nothing like I have had in the past but I am still having to go to the bathroom 10-15 times a day. When I have a gas attack I feel like I have to have a BM (tenesmus). Many times I go to the bathroom and nothing happens. I get tired of that so I hold off on going to the bathroom and inevitably I have an accident. I still wear Depends Real Fit. They are great and have never let me down. It sucks but that is my reality these days.

I want to improve so much more. I don't want this urgency. I don't want the gas attacks. What should I do now? The 10 days of FMT really did a lot. I am not on any meds. I think the next step is 10 more days of transplants. Dr. Bansidhar wants me to get another colonoscopy in August. I will hold off until summer is over. I want him to see that I am cured so I need to plan for another round of FMT soon. I am not looking forward to that but what options do I have? I want my life back dammit!

7/7/2014

I had a really nice Fourth of July weekend and didn't have many problems. My system seems to be functioning properly even though the damage is still evident. I am processing food well and gaining nutrients. My BMs are formed though I still have wetness. I have gas attacks still and feel some urgency but all in all I am much better than I was last year at this time. I was able to swim in the pool with the grandkids without worrying about having an accident. Last year I put a bucket in the garage just in case of an emergency. I never used it but I had it available.

I started exercising 3 weeks ago and managed to go 2 weeks, 4 days per week. I was doing stretches, pushups, crunches, rowing, toe touches, weight lifting and a few other light exercises. I stopped last Monday because of stiffness in my back. I have been walking and riding my bike daily also. I plan to start a light routine tomorrow. I do it easy to get in the habit. I will start at 10 reps and work my way back up to 50, that's where I was before I got sick.

I am going to the bathroom a lot. I feel like I have to go bad but often when I sit down I don't produce much. Up until recently I would have to go every time I started to eat. That has stopped and I can now go to a restaurant and eat a meal and not have to excuse myself. That is awesome!

I did an experiment and ate 2 cream filled Dolly Madison chocolate cupcakes from the machine here at work last week. I know it was foolish but I was so hungry! That evening I had D and was up a lot throughout the night. I suffered for a couple days with gas and actually thought I was going to flare. My system settled down then and I went back to normal. No more super sweet junk foods for me! I am able drink a beer or two without noticing any changes. I enjoy that. I also noticed that when I have a few vodka and tonics on Saturday night that on Sunday my BMs are more solid. I decided to try 2 shots of vodka medicinally before bed to see if it would help my system. It didn't really do anything but make me more tired in the morning. I am quitting that. I tried some coconut water last week but got D from that. My wife read that it was real good for the digestion among other things. I think I drank too much and am going to try it again this week in smaller quantities.

I keep looking for something that will help me step up to the next level. I have gained some footing this past month and feel better. I feel hopeful that I will continue to improve and someday be normal again. Well, as normal as I can be!

8/5/2014

Here we are in August already. Holy shit this summer is going by fast! We have had a lot of rain here in Erie, PA and it has been an unseasonably cool summer but I have enjoyed it very much. That's because I don't have Ulcerative Colitis anymore and I am feeling great! Through the first weeks of July I was still very gassy and had a lot of wetness. I felt myself getting better the past week and today I feel wonderful! I have been going less and feel much more energetic. It's like I have been taking little tiny baby steps and suddenly took a big step! I don't know what caused that but I know it's good. My gas is way less and I am not running to the bathroom all day long. I can eat and drink what I want (including extreme sweets like cake) without any problems. I am sleeping well and enjoying doing all the things I used to do before I got sick. My wife and I don't talk crap anymore either. When it was consuming my life it seemed to be all we talked about. I am loving this!

I started taking an iron supplement (Gentle Iron) last week. Maybe that has helped me step up. I had to start taking Omeprazole for my heartburn on Sunday. I tried everything and was starting to take too many

Tums again so I decided it was necessary to medicate. After only 3 days I am heartburn free. I think the H2 blocker is better than the Proton Pump inhibitor. I wasn't having Gerd, I was getting burning low in my stomach and was afraid I might be getting an ulcer. I will let you know how it goes with this. I really don't like taking medicine for long term. It was getting so annoying that I had no choice. It pisses me off that my flexible spending plan will not pay for over the counter meds. That's just wrong!

I started taking a protein drink in the morning again. I had some leftover Warrior Force so I figured I might as well use it up. I wanted to boost my Albumen levels again now that I am not having diarrhea to allow my body to repair the damaged tissue in my colon. It seems to be helping. I also started exercising again. I like the way I feel after a light workout. I haven't been riding my bike much. I have to start doing that again. Winter isn't that far off.

I still wear the adult diapers but am planning to stop those soon. I only had one small accident last month so I think it's time to start thinking about giving that security blanket up. I hate wearing a diaper in the summer. It's so hot and irritating. I remember when I was a kid thinking about how some old people have to wear a diaper and how weak they must be. Like it was something they wanted. I am the old man now. It sucks. It's embarrassing and I can't wait until I can live without them!

Dr. Bansidhars' office has sent me some reminders 'time for your colonoscopy'. I thought it over seriously and have decided not to get another one. It's invasive and can cause a lot of problems. I feel great and am healing nicely and don't want to do anything to disturb my progress. He worries about me getting cancer but I am not worried. I guess I don't have any faith in him or any doctors. I know he cares but I think he may be brainwashed by the system. He wants to make money, he needs to make a lot of money to continue his practice. I am not saying he is just in it for the money but it is a reality in the world we live in. I am going to take my chances and hope for the best. If I didn't have to pay so much for insurance and flexible spending I could retire much earlier. It sucks. I pay so much but don't want to go to the doctor. I don't think they can help with chronic illness. I keep my insurance for major medical emergencies. That's it.

That's all for now. The fecal transplant worked for me. If you are like me and want to get back to normal I suggest you give it a try. You have nothing to lose and everything to gain. It's not that bad and I am very glad I did it. Life is fun again!

8/25/2014

I have been going without adult diapers for 2 weeks now and things are going well. I have not had any accidents. I do wear them when I go somewhere and am not sure if there will be a bathroom. I have gained a lot of confidence and soon won't have to wear them at all. That is huge!

I wanted to correct something from my last post. I said I was cured of Ulcerative Colitis but I am still seeing some blood even though I don't have diarrhea or urgency and have been making solids for a while now. I don't know if the blood is from a damaged colon or if I still have ulcerations. I only see a small amount of bright red blood after I go in the morning and usually only on Monday morning. Usually I make a nice solid and go a lot and then see the blood when I wipe. I also have some wetness still and sometimes make small white raisins. I also see white streaks in the solids sometimes. It's weird. I know I am doing much better and have resumed living my life. I guess I need to have a colonoscopy and let the doctor tell me I don't have U.C.anymore before I can make that statement with assurance.

That's all I wanted to say for now. I am doing well and I truly believe that fecal transplant is the answer.

10/28/2014

It's been a couple months since I wrote so I wanted to give an update. I had an amazing weekend. Went to see the Canadian rock band Big Wreck at the Town Ballroom in Buffalo on Saturday. Had a huge dinner at the Bijou including salad with my favorite dressing - blue cheese, caponatina for an appetizer, a couple of Labatt Blues (bottle), chicken pot pie for the entre', and apple crisp with vanilla ice cream for dessert. I do not miss the SCD at all! I have had a bad cold for a couple weeks and am not completely over it but I enjoyed the show anyways. It's so great to be able to go out again!

Here's where I am at in my healing. I am having less bowel movements, averaging about 5 per day. I have found that draft beer really does upset my system where bottled or canned does not so I am avoiding that. I still see a tiny bit of blood from time to time and have some wetness but that seems to be lessening. I am much less gassy and my BMs do not smell that bad. I quit the adult diapers completely and have not had any accidents. I can actually hold it for a while and am beginning to get over the panicky feeling. I am taking Omeprazole. I have tried so many things for heartburn and some actually helped but the main issue is that I get it when I am doing something physical. I need instant relief and do not want to take Tums so I am staying on the H2 blocker for now. Maybe someday I can figure that out too. I take an Iron supplement and a B vitamin daily. I am exercising 4 days a week in the morning. I walk at lunchtime, a little over a mile. My knees feel better but I have some pain in the joints. It's not as much pain as discomfort and I still have the feeling that my knee might buckle if I kick my leg out too far when I'm walking. I feel improvement but it's a slow, slow process. My weight has leveled off at 191 and I think that is perfect for me (I am 5'10" tall). I was using Aussie Freeze on my hair (I have long hair) to keep it from looking crazy but noticed that I was losing a lot. I clean the shower drain every Friday and was removing a lot of hair out of it. I changed from that product to Argan Oil and in the past few weeks noticed a dramatic lessening of hair in the drain. My wife told me that the Aussie wasn't good for my hair and she was right again!

I have many random thoughts about what I have been through and sometimes feel very angry at a medical system that let me get so damaged inside. Healing the colon is like trying to heal a broken leg while jogging. It's a slow, painful, almost impossible process. If I had gotten proper treatment and a fecal transplant sooner I would be totally cured by now. If you think about it we are all pretty much screwed. I have decent insurance (I pay $250 deductible and 20% of the total which I think is bullshit!) so the incentive for the medical community is for me to have expensive surgery and/or meds. If I get better they make nothing. I believe that doctors would want to help but they are blocked by the insurance companies and by fear of being sued. I would like to find a doctor that I could pay cash. I would even pay him a yearly retainer fee. I pay $80 a week for insurance and I have $40 a week taken out for my flex plan. That's over $6000 a year and I am afraid to go to the doctor! I am afraid that they will look at me and see dollar signs! I would be willing to bet that there are doctors who are getting tired of this system and would consider taking a limited number of patients on retainer and a cash basis only. Drop the insurance, promise not to sue and form a trusting relationship. That's possible!

12/4/2014

I had a very nice Thanksgiving holiday. I didn't stuff myself but it was nice to be able to eat anything I wanted without fear of flaring. I am healing and getting better every day. When I think back to how I was a year ago I am amazed! I feel normal again. I am losing the fear of having an accident because I can hold it now. I have held it for an hour! No more panicking, no more diapers, no more Ulcerative Colitis. I am seriously considering going without medical insurance. People think I'm crazy when I say that. What I think is crazy is paying into a system that wants me to stay sick. I don't want their drugs. I don't need them telling there is no cure for my condition or that I am a defective person. I don't live extravagantly by any means but I cannot afford insurance anymore. I am in debt and it is getting worse. I need that 6K!

2/3/2015

Had a wonderful Christmas and a nice quiet New Years. My health is improving even though I have continued to have some wetness and a small amount of blood when I wipe some mornings. I believe this is due to the extent of the damage that occurred while I was flaring. If I had one word of advice to give to people about U.C. it would be to not wait until it gets so bad that you have to be hospitalized like I did. It seems that once you get so severely damaged you may never heal completely. One thing that prompted me to write today is a major improvement I have had recently. I quit drinking flavored vodka and tonic water and my gas has gone way down. I have solids every day. I also noticed that fruit seems to make me gassy as well so I keep it to a minimum. I can eat and drink anything but I have noticed some foods cause slight reactions, mainly gas. With the wetness I sometimes experience, gas can be a problem (can you say sharts!). I gained another pound and now weigh 194. I have been exercising and my previous energy level has returned. It's great to be able to do things again without worrying about where the bathroom is. I still get nervous when I have gas but am doing so much better. It takes a long time to heal physically and mentally. I am so glad that I did the fecal transplant. I decided to cancel my medical insurance. My wife agreed and had me cancel hers too. I was a bit nervous but we made it through January and we're both still alive and doing well. There is a sense of freedom when you know that if you need a doctor he won't be looking at how much you are worth. My father didn't trust doctors. He isn't on any meds and just had his 85th Birthday! There are good doctors and there are times when you need a doctor. The for-profit medical system in this country is wrong and we all know it. Can it be changed? I don't know but as an act of civil disobedience I protest being forced to pay into a system that I do not value or trust.

3/23/2015

I am convinced that I am cured. I have not had any major set-backs since I began this process. There have been times of doubt but I haven't flared. I took another step up in my health recently and I attribute that to changing my work schedule and possibly the hemp protein I began taking in the evenings. I feel very happy these days. I am getting back into my music and my energy levels are almost back to normal. I continue to heal seeing very little blood and having less and less urgency. I haven't had any prolonged diarrhea since I did the transplants. I do not wear adult diapers on a regular basis anymore. I only wear them when I am traveling or someplace where a bathroom is unavailable. I highly recommend this therapy. It has been amazing to have my life back. I just wish I didn't have so much damage done to my system. It could have been avoided had I known about FMT sooner. I blame the doctors for that.

4/21/2015

I quit drinking draft beer completely since I was having a lot of gas. I didn't want to blame it on beer but since I stopped drinking it my gas has gone way down. I always enjoyed beer but have switched to Twisted Tea. It's pretty good and doesn't bother me at all. I continue to heal albeit very slowly. It's weird though but because of the damage to my colon when I have to go I feel like I have to go now (tenesmus again). I can hold it but as I walk to the bathroom I feel this nervousness and anxiety like I'm not going to make it. It's psychological damage. I don't have accidents anymore but I still have anxiety. I think this will eventually go away but it takes so damn long. Things are going good and I have no fear of relapse. FMT was the answer for me.

4/5/2016

I am cured! It's been almost a year since I last wrote and the healing has continued. I bought a new guitar recently and have been playing again and am getting back to songwriting. I have had my energy return and UC is no longer a part of my daily life. I feel wonderful and this experience had made me so grateful for my health. I eat and drink anything I want, I don't have any more symptoms and I am living again. I hope my story has helped you to have hope. I want you to be cured as I was. Do what needs to be done and get back to living!

A Final Word

There is so much more I would like to say about what I have been through but I think a few main thoughts will be enough. The feeling of helplessness you get when you are diagnosed with an incurable chronic illness is absolutely terrifying! I spent 10 years, all of my fifties on this! I will be 60 this coming Sunday May 29th and there is only one way I can see any good coming from what I suffered. That is to help others. When I hear stories of people, especially children who have been diagnosed with bowel disease I feel so sad. To think of their lives being put on hold or maybe even ended by a condition that is totally and easily curable just makes me want to cry. A person who has not suffered with this cannot begin to comprehend its horrible reality. We go to the bathroom and forget it. We take its simplicity for granted. Imagine getting up every half hour after going to bed at night, imagine lying in bed so tired and worn out that you can hardly move but still you have to get up because otherwise you might have an accident. Imagine being in the shower and having an attack. Trying to drive to work or just make it to Country Fair. Imagine not being able to make it and pooping in your underwear while you're driving. Imagine your wife or husband sitting in the car with you suffering the smell and the inconvenience of having to turn around and drive back home. You cannot make any plans. Imagine not being able to go anywhere without knowing if there is a bathroom available. You are at a restaurant and find that the single stall bathroom is occupied. You are at work and have an emergency and the restroom is full, you make it to another restroom and it is occupied also. You have an accident at work! You make it home and are so tired, bleeding, but the lawn needs mowed or the snow cleared from the driveway. You are starving but do not want to eat. The pain in your belly feels like an angry weasel is living in there. You call the doctor and they tell you to take some Imodium. You live moment to moment in terror. You feel like you have to go but are not sure. You try and nothing happens. How long do you sit on the toilet and wait? You finally give up and leave the restroom but you feel like you have to go again. You are home watching TV with your loved one and five minutes into the show you have to go to the bathroom, fifteen minutes later you try again but you still feel like you have to go. You wither away little by little until nothing is left. You end up hospitalized with only one option. Removal of your Colon. Even after that you can have serious problems. You can even continue to have U.C.! This shit has changed me forever. Sure I can joke about it. I am living proof that U.C. is curable! I am strong again! I am healthy and living fearlessly. Life is good and I am glad that god didn't answer my prayers. I asked him to let me die. I begged him! I don't even believe in a traditional god and yet I pleaded with him to take me. I hope to get back to making some new music soon. This time I am going to write songs that are happy. Songs of love and hope. Songs that inspire and strengthen. Yes I am happy to be alive. Happy 60th Birthday to Me!